LOW FODMAP COOKBOOK FOR BEGINNERS:

1200+ Simple and Delicious Recipes to Calm Your Guts and Combat Digestive Issues

BY

NELSON ROBINSON

TABLE OF CONTENTS

INTRODUCTION

In recent years, the Low FODMAP diet has gained significant attention and recognition as a therapeutic approach to managing digestive discomfort and symptoms associated with irritable bowel syndrome (IBS) and other gastrointestinal disorders. FODMAPs, an acronym for Fermentable Oligosaccharides, Disaccharides, Monosaccharides, and Polyols, are a group of short-chain carbohydrates and sugar alcohols that can trigger digestive distress in susceptible individuals.

The Low FODMAP diet was developed by researchers at Monash University in Melbourne, Australia, and has become a widely adopted dietary strategy for those seeking relief from bloating, gas, abdominal pain, and irregular bowel movements. The core concept of the Low FODMAP diet involves reducing the intake of certain types of carbohydrates that are poorly absorbed in the small intestine, leading to fermentation and gas production in the colon.

Cooking plays a pivotal role in successfully adhering to the Low FODMAP diet, as it requires careful consideration of ingredient choices, portion sizes, and cooking techniques. Creating delicious and satisfying meals within the constraints of the Low FODMAP framework may initially seem challenging, but with the right knowledge and creativity, one can discover a diverse range of flavorful and nourishing options.

In this culinary journey, individuals embarking on the Low FODMAP diet can explore a plethora of whole, unprocessed foods that are naturally low in FODMAPs. Ingredients such as lean proteins, gluten-free grains, certain fruits and vegetables, and lactose-free dairy products become the foundation for crafting appetizing meals. The challenge lies in finding alternative sources of flavor, texture, and complexity to compensate for the restriction of high-FODMAP ingredients like garlic, onions, and certain spices.

Herbs, spices, and other Low FODMAP flavor enhancers become essential allies in the Low FODMAP kitchen, allowing individuals to infuse their dishes with aromatic profiles that mimic traditional recipes. Experimentation with garlic-infused oils, chives, and infused vinegars becomes a skill to be honed, transforming the cooking process into a culinary adventure.

Furthermore, understanding portion sizes and moderation is crucial in maintaining a balanced and well-rounded Low FODMAP diet. While some foods may be low in FODMAPs in smaller quantities, consuming excessive amounts could lead to an accumulation of fermentable carbohydrates, potentially triggering symptoms. A well-rounded plate that includes a variety of nutrient-dense ingredients is key to ensuring optimal health while adhering to the Low FODMAP guidelines.

As we delve deeper into the world of Low FODMAP diet cooking, this journey is not just about restriction; it is about discovering a new appreciation for the richness of whole foods and the artistry of crafting flavorful meals within the constraints of dietary guidelines. With a thoughtful and creative approach to cooking, individuals can not only manage their digestive symptoms but also savor a diverse and satisfying array of dishes that celebrate the nourishing power of food tailored to their unique needs.

CHAPTER 1: WELCOME TO THE LOW FODMAP LIFESTYLE

Understanding FODMAPs and Digestive Health

If you've ever experienced digestive discomfort, bloating, or abdominal pain, you're not alone. Many individuals grapple with digestive issues that can significantly impact their quality of life. Enter the Low FODMAP Lifestyle – a revolutionary approach to managing digestive health that has gained popularity in recent years.

FODMAPs, which stands for Fermentable Oligosaccharides, Disaccharides, Monosaccharides, and Polyols, are a group of carbohydrates found in certain foods that can be poorly absorbed in the small intestine. The malabsorption of these compounds can lead to fermentation by gut bacteria, resulting in symptoms such as gas, bloating, abdominal pain, and altered bowel habits. The Low FODMAP Diet, developed by researchers at Monash University in Australia, aims to identify and eliminate high-FODMAP foods from one's diet to alleviate digestive symptoms.

Understanding FODMAPs:
Fermentable: These carbohydrates are easily fermented by bacteria in the gut, leading to gas production and bloating.

Oligosaccharides: Found in foods like wheat, rye, onions, and garlic, these short-chain carbohydrates can be challenging for some individuals to digest.

Disaccharides: Lactose, a sugar present in dairy products, falls under this category. People with lactose intolerance may experience digestive issues when consuming high-lactose foods.

Monosaccharides: Fructose, a natural sugar found in fruits, honey, and some sweeteners, can cause digestive discomfort in sensitive individuals.

Polyols: Sugar alcohols like sorbitol and mannitol, present in certain fruits, vegetables, and artificial sweeteners, can be poorly absorbed and lead to bloating.

Embarking on the Low FODMAP Lifestyle:

Elimination Phase: The first step involves removing high-FODMAP foods from your diet for a specified period (usually 2-6 weeks). This phase helps identify trigger foods and provides relief from digestive symptoms.

Reintroduction Phase: After the elimination phase, high-FODMAP foods are gradually reintroduced one at a time to pinpoint specific triggers. This phase is personalized, allowing individuals to understand their unique tolerance levels.

Maintenance Phase: Armed with knowledge about their FODMAP triggers, individuals can adopt a sustainable, balanced diet that accommodates their digestive needs. It's crucial to maintain a varied and nutritionally adequate diet while avoiding specific trigger foods.

Benefits of the Low FODMAP Lifestyle:

Symptom Relief: Many individuals experience significant relief from symptoms such as bloating, gas, and abdominal pain.

Improved Quality of Life: Managing digestive symptoms can lead to enhanced well-being, increased energy levels, and improved daily functioning.

Personalized Approach: The Low FODMAP Lifestyle is not a one-size-fits-all solution. It is tailored to each individual's unique tolerances and preferences.

Scientific Backing: The diet is backed by extensive research conducted by Monash University, providing a solid foundation for its efficacy.

In conclusion, the Low FODMAP Lifestyle offers a promising path to digestive well-being. By understanding FODMAPs and their impact on the digestive system, individuals can take control of their health and make informed choices to create a sustainable, satisfying, and symptom-free lifestyle. Always consult with a healthcare professional or a registered dietitian before making significant dietary changes, especially if you have pre-existing health conditions. Welcome to a journey of discovery and empowerment on the road to digestive health!

Getting Started: Stocking Your Low FODMAP Kitchen

Embarking on the Low FODMAP lifestyle is a transformative journey for individuals seeking relief from gastrointestinal discomfort and seeking to improve their overall well-being. FODMAPs, which stands for Fermentable Oligosaccharides, Disaccharides, Monosaccharides, and Polyols, are a group of short-chain carbohydrates that can trigger digestive symptoms in some people.

Getting started on the Low FODMAP lifestyle begins with setting up a well-stocked kitchen that supports your dietary needs. Here's a comprehensive guide to help you navigate the process:

Understanding Low FODMAP Foods:

Before diving into stocking your kitchen, it's essential to familiarize yourself with Low FODMAP foods. These include fruits like berries, oranges, and grapes; vegetables like spinach, carrots, and bell peppers; proteins such as chicken, beef, and tofu; and grains like rice and quinoa. Additionally, lactose-free dairy and certain nuts and seeds are often Low FODMAP.

Kitchen Staples Checklist:

Low FODMAP Vegetables: Stock up on zucchini, cucumber, carrots, spinach, kale, and other low FODMAP vegetables. These will serve as the foundation for many meals.

Low FODMAP Fruits: Opt for berries, oranges, grapes, and bananas in moderation.

These fruits can be enjoyed as snacks or incorporated into meals.

Proteins: Choose lean proteins like chicken, turkey, beef, fish, and tofu. Eggs are also a great option.

Lactose-Free Dairy: If you tolerate dairy, select lactose-free options such as lactose-free milk, hard cheeses, and lactose-free yogurt.

Grains: Fill your pantry with gluten-free grains like rice, quinoa, oats, and corn. These will be the base for many of your meals.

Herbs and Spices: Flavor your dishes with herbs like basil, oregano, thyme, and spices such as cumin and paprika. Avoid onion and garlic-based seasonings.

FODMAP-Friendly Condiments: Choose condiments like mustard, mayonnaise, and vinegar without high FODMAP ingredients.

Low FODMAP Sweeteners: Opt for sweeteners like maple syrup, rice malt syrup, and certain artificial sweeteners like sucralose or stevia.

Gluten-Free Products: For those sensitive to gluten, explore gluten-free alternatives such as gluten-free bread, pasta, and flour.

Nuts and Seeds: Include almonds, walnuts, chia seeds, and flaxseeds in your kitchen. Be cautious with high FODMAP options like cashews and pistachios.

Meal Planning and Preparation:

Create a Meal Plan: Planning your meals in advance helps ensure you have all the necessary ingredients on hand and reduces the likelihood of accidentally consuming high FODMAP foods.

Batch Cooking: Prepare meals in batches to save time during the week. This can be particularly helpful when dealing with a busy schedule.

Experiment with Recipes: Explore Low FODMAP recipes to add variety to your meals. There are numerous creative and delicious options that cater to your dietary needs.

Seek Guidance:

If you're new to the Low FODMAP lifestyle, consider consulting with a registered dietitian or healthcare professional who specializes in gastrointestinal health. They can provide personalized guidance based on your individual needs and help you navigate the complexities of the diet.

Embarking on the Low FODMAP lifestyle is a step towards better digestive health, and a well-stocked kitchen is your ally in this journey. By carefully selecting Low FODMAP foods and incorporating them into delicious and nutritious meals, you can optimize your well-being and enjoy a more comfortable, symptom-free lifestyle.

Basics ingredients of low fodmap cooking

If you've been grappling with digestive issues, you're not alone. The Low FODMAP lifestyle might be the key to unlocking a new chapter of digestive wellness for you. FODMAPs, which stands for Fermentable Oligosaccharides, Disaccharides, Monosaccharides, and Polyols, are a group of short-chain carbohydrates that can trigger digestive discomfort in some individuals.

Adopting the Low FODMAP lifestyle involves navigating through a variety of foods to identify and eliminate potential triggers. However, fear not! The journey is not about deprivation; it's about discovering delicious alternatives that suit your digestive needs. Let's dive into the basics of low FODMAP cooking and explore some essential ingredients to get you started on this transformative culinary adventure.

1. Proteins: Lean and Clean

Opt for lean proteins such as chicken, turkey, fish, eggs, and tofu. These sources provide essential nutrients without the added FODMAPs found in certain cuts of meat.

2. Vegetables: Choose Wisely

Stick to low FODMAP vegetables like carrots, zucchini, bell peppers, and spinach. These add color, flavor, and essential nutrients to your meals without causing digestive distress.

3. Fruits: Sweet and Safe

Enjoy fruits with lower FODMAP content, including strawberries, blueberries, oranges, and kiwi. Be mindful of portion sizes to keep

FODMAP intake within the recommended limits.

4. Grains: Go Gluten-Free

Embrace gluten-free grains like rice, quinoa, and oats. These grains provide a satisfying base for your meals while steering clear of high FODMAP culprits.

5. Dairy: Lactose-Free Delights

Opt for lactose-free or low-lactose dairy products like lactose-free milk, hard cheeses, and lactose-free yogurt. These alternatives ensure that you still enjoy the creamy goodness without compromising your digestive comfort.

6. Fats and Oils: Healthy Choices

Incorporate healthy fats and oils such as olive oil, coconut oil, and butter (without lactose).

These add richness and flavor to your dishes without contributing to FODMAP-related discomfort.

7. Herbs and Spices: Flavor Explosion

Jazz up your meals with low FODMAP herbs and spices like basil, thyme, rosemary, and ginger. These not only enhance the taste but also offer potential digestive benefits.

8. Sweeteners: Mindful Indulgences

Opt for sweeteners like maple syrup, golden syrup, or stevia. Be cautious with portion sizes and explore moderation in sweetness to maintain a low FODMAP balance.

Remember, the key to success in the Low FODMAP lifestyle is balance and variety. Experiment with different ingredients, try new recipes, and pay attention to your body's responses. It's a journey of self-discovery that can lead to a happier, healthier digestive system. So, welcome to the Low FODMAP lifestyle — where delicious and digestive-friendly meals await!

CHAPTER 2: BREAKFAST DELIGHTS

Scrambled Egg and Spinach Muffins

Time Frame:

Prep Time: 10 minutes

Cook Time: 20 minutes

Total Time: 30 minutes

Ingredients:

1. *6 large eggs*
2. *1 cup chopped spinach*
3. *1/2 cup diced bell peppers*
4. *1/4 cup shredded cheese*
5. *Salt and pepper to taste*
6. *Cooking spray*

Instructions:

1. *Preheat the oven to 350°F (175°C) and grease a muffin tin with cooking spray.*
2. *In a bowl, whisk together eggs, spinach, bell peppers, cheese, salt, and pepper.*
3. *Pour the egg mixture into the muffin cups, filling each about 2/3 full.*
4. *Bake for 15-20 minutes or until the eggs are set.*
5. *Allow the muffins to cool slightly before serving.*

Tips:

1. *Customize with your favorite vegetables or add cooked bacon for extra flavor.*
2. *Make a batch ahead for quick breakfasts throughout the week.*

Blueberry Banana Pancakes

Time Frame:

Prep Time: 15 minutes

Cook Time: 10 minutes

Total Time: 25 minutes

Ingredients:

1. *1 cup all-purpose flour*
2. *1 tablespoon sugar*
3. *1 teaspoon baking powder*
4. *1/2 teaspoon baking soda*
5. *1/4 teaspoon salt*
6. *1 cup buttermilk*
7. *1 ripe banana, mashed*
8. *1/2 cup blueberries*
9. *Butter or oil for cooking*

Instructions:

1. *In a bowl, whisk together flour, sugar, baking powder, baking soda, and salt.*

2. *In another bowl, mix buttermilk and mashed banana.*

3. *Add the wet ingredients to the dry ingredients and stir until just combined. Fold in the blueberries.*

4. *Heat a griddle or skillet over medium heat and grease with butter or oil.*

5. *Pour 1/4 cup of batter onto the griddle for each pancake. Cook until bubbles form on the surface, then flip and cook until golden brown.*

Tips:

1. Serve with maple syrup, yogurt, or additional fresh fruit.

2. Double the batch and freeze extra pancakes for busy mornings.

Quinoa Breakfast Bowl with Maple Pecans

Time Frame:

Prep Time: 10 minutes

Cook Time: 15 minutes

Total Time: 25 minutes

Ingredients:

1. *1 cup cooked quinoa*

2. *1/4 cup chopped pecans*

3. *1 tablespoon maple syrup*

4. *1/2 cup Greek yogurt*

5. *Fresh berries for topping*

Instructions:

1. *In a small pan, toast pecans over medium heat until fragrant.*

2. *Add maple syrup to the pan and stir until pecans are coated. Remove from heat.*

3. *In a bowl, layer cooked quinoa, maple pecans, Greek yogurt, and fresh berries.*

Tips:

1. *Experiment with different nuts or seeds for added crunch.*
2. *Drizzle additional maple syrup for extra sweetness.*

Chia Seed Pudding with Kiwi Slices

Time Frame:

Prep Time: 5 minutes

Chill Time: 2 hours (or overnight)

Total Time: 2 hours 5 minutes

Ingredients:

1. *1/4 cup chia seeds*
2. *1 cup almond milk (or any milk of choice)*
3. *1 tablespoon honey or maple syrup*
4. *Kiwi slices for topping*

Instructions:

1. *In a jar or bowl, mix chia seeds, almond milk, and sweetener.*
2. *Stir well and refrigerate for at least 2 hours or overnight, allowing the chia seeds to absorb the liquid.*

3. *Before serving, stir the pudding and top with kiwi slices.*

Tips:

1. *Add vanilla extract or cinnamon for extra flavor.*
2. *Customize with your favorite fruit toppings.*

Turkey and Vegetable Omelette

Time Frame:

Prep Time: 10 minutes

Cook Time: 10 minutes

Total Time: 20 minutes

Ingredients:

1. *3 large eggs*
2. *1/4 cup diced turkey*
3. *1/4 cup diced bell peppers*
4. *1/4 cup diced onions*
5. *1/4 cup shredded cheese*
6. *Salt and pepper to taste*
7. *Olive oil for cooking*

Instructions:

1. *In a bowl, beat the eggs and season with salt and pepper.*

2. *Heat olive oil in a non-stick skillet over medium heat.*

3. *Add turkey, bell peppers, and onions to the skillet. Cook until vegetables are tender.*

4. *Pour beaten eggs over the vegetables, tilting the pan to spread them evenly.*

5. *Once the edges set, sprinkle shredded cheese on one half of the omelette and fold the other half over the cheese. Cook until the cheese melts.*

Tips:

1. *Use leftover cooked vegetables or meats for a quicker omelette.*

2. *Garnish with fresh herbs or salsa for added flavor.*

Smoothie Bowl with Low FODMAP Fruits

Time Frame:

Prep Time: 5 minutes

Total Time: 5 minutes

Ingredients:

1. *1 cup low FODMAP fruits (e.g., berries, kiwi, banana)*
2. *1/2 cup lactose-free yogurt*
3. *1/4 cup gluten-free granola*
4. *1 tablespoon chia seeds*
5. *Ice cubes (optional)*

Instructions:

1. *Blend low FODMAP fruits and yogurt until smooth. Add ice cubes if desired.*
2. *Pour the smoothie into a bowl.*

3. *Top with gluten-free granola and chia seeds.*

Tips:

1. *Choose fruits that are low in FODMAPs, such as berries, kiwi, and banana.*

2. *Customize with additional toppings like shredded coconut or sliced almonds.*

3. *Enjoy your delicious and nutritious breakfast options!*

CHAPTER 3: LUNCHTIME FAVORITES

Grilled Chicken and Avocado Salad

Time Frame:

Prep Time: 15 minutes

Cook Time: 10 minutes

Total Time: 25 minutes

Ingredients:

1. *1 lb boneless, skinless chicken breasts*
2. *Salt and pepper to taste*
3. *6 cups mixed salad greens*
4. *1 cup cherry tomatoes, halved*
5. *1 avocado, sliced*
6. *1/4 cup red onion, thinly sliced*
7. *1/4 cup feta cheese, crumbled*

8. Balsamic vinaigrette dressing

Instructions:

1. *Season chicken breasts with salt and pepper, then grill until fully cooked.*
2. *Let the chicken rest for a few minutes, then slice it into strips.*
3. *In a large bowl, combine salad greens, cherry tomatoes, avocado, red onion, and grilled chicken.*
4. *Drizzle with balsamic vinaigrette and toss gently.*
5. *Top with crumbled feta cheese before serving.*

Tips:

1. *Customize with additional vegetables or nuts for extra crunch.*

2. Use your favorite dressing or make a homemade vinaigrette.

Quinoa and Vegetable Stuffed Peppers

Time Frame:

Prep Time: 20 minutes

Cook Time: 30 minutes

Total Time: 50 minutes

Ingredients:

1. *4 bell peppers, halved and seeds removed*
2. *1 cup cooked quinoa*
3. *1 cup black beans, drained and rinsed*
4. *1 cup corn kernels*
5. *1 cup diced tomatoes*
6. *1 cup shredded cheddar cheese*
7. *1 teaspoon cumin*
8. *1 teaspoon chili powder*
9. *Salt and pepper to taste*
10. *Fresh cilantro for garnish*

Instructions:

1. *Preheat the oven to 375°F (190°C).*

2. *In a bowl, combine cooked quinoa, black beans, corn, tomatoes, cheese, cumin, chili powder, salt, and pepper.*

3. *Stuff each pepper half with the quinoa mixture.*

4. *Place stuffed peppers in a baking dish and bake for 25-30 minutes or until peppers are tender.*

5. *Garnish with fresh cilantro before serving.*

Tips:

1. *Add ground meat or tofu to the quinoa mixture for extra protein.*

2. *Serve with a dollop of Greek yogurt or salsa.*

Zucchini Noodles with Pesto and Cherry Tomatoes

Time Frame:

Prep Time: 15 minutes

Cook Time: 5 minutes

Total Time: 20 minutes

Ingredients:

1. *4 medium-sized zucchini, spiralized into noodles*
2. *1 cup cherry tomatoes, halved*
3. *1/2 cup basil pesto*
4. *1/4 cup pine nuts, toasted*
5. *Parmesan cheese for garnish*

Instructions:

1. *In a large pan, sauté zucchini noodles over medium heat for 3-5 minutes or until just tender.*

2. *Add cherry tomatoes to the pan and toss for an additional 1-2 minutes.*

3. *Stir in the basil pesto and toss until the noodles are well coated.*

4. *Transfer to a serving dish, sprinkle with toasted pine nuts, and garnish with Parmesan cheese.*

Tips:

1. *Make your own pesto or use store-bought for convenience.*

2. *Top with grilled chicken or shrimp for a complete meal.*

Salmon and Cucumber Sushi Rolls

Time Frame:

Prep Time: 30 minutes

Cook Time: 0 minutes (assuming using smoked or cooked salmon)

Total Time: 30 minutes

Ingredients:

1. *2 cups sushi rice, cooked and seasoned*
2. *4 nori seaweed sheets*
3. *1/2 pound smoked or cooked salmon, sliced*
4. *1 cucumber, julienned*
5. *Soy sauce and wasabi for serving*
6. *Pickled ginger for garnish*

Instructions:

1. *Place a nori sheet on a bamboo sushi rolling mat.*

2. *Spread a thin layer of sushi rice over the nori, leaving a border at the top.*

3. *Arrange slices of salmon and julienned cucumber along the bottom edge of the rice.*

4. *Roll the sushi tightly from the bottom, using the bamboo mat as a guide.*

5. *Seal the edge with a little water and slice the roll into bite-sized pieces.*

6. *Serve with soy sauce, wasabi, and pickled ginger.*

Tips:

1. *Experiment with different fillings like avocado or cream cheese.*

2. *Use a sharp knife to ensure clean cuts when slicing the rolls.*

Greek-style Chicken Wrap with Tzatziki

Time Frame:

Prep Time: 20 minutes

Cook Time: 10 minutes

Total Time: 30 minutes

Ingredients:

1. *1 lb boneless, skinless chicken breasts, grilled and sliced*
2. *4 whole-grain wraps*
3. *1 cup cherry tomatoes, halved*
4. *1 cucumber, sliced*
5. *1/2 red onion, thinly sliced*
6. *Feta cheese, crumbled*
7. *Tzatziki sauce*

Instructions:

1. *Lay out the wraps and evenly distribute the sliced chicken among them.*
2. *Add cherry tomatoes, cucumber slices, red onion, and crumbled feta to each wrap.*
3. *Drizzle tzatziki sauce over the fillings.*
4. *Fold in the sides of the wraps and roll them up.*

Tips:

1. *Warm the wraps before assembling for a softer texture.*
2. *Add Kalamata olives or hummus for extra Mediterranean flavor.*

Tomato Basil Soup with Parmesan Crisps

Time Frame:

Prep Time: 15 minutes

Cook Time: 30 minutes

Total Time: 45 minutes

Ingredients:

1. *1 tablespoon olive oil*

2. *1 onion, chopped*

3. *2 cloves garlic, minced*

4. *2 cans (28 oz each) whole tomatoes, crushed*

5. *1 cup vegetable broth*

6. *1/2 cup fresh basil, chopped*

7. *Salt and pepper to taste*

8. *1 cup heavy cream (optional)*

9. *Parmesan crisps for garnish*

Instructions:

1. *In a large pot, heat olive oil over medium heat. Add chopped onion and garlic, sauté until softened.*

2. *Pour in crushed tomatoes and vegetable broth. Bring to a simmer.*

3. *Stir in fresh basil and season with salt and pepper. Simmer for 20-25 minutes.*

4. *If desired, blend the soup until smooth using an immersion blender or countertop blender.*

5. *Stir in heavy cream (if using) and heat through.*

6. *Serve the soup hot, garnished with Parmesan crisps.*

Tips:

1. *Make the Parmesan crisps by baking small piles of grated Parmesan cheese until crispy.*

2. *For a lighter version, omit the cream and use a drizzle of olive oil on top.*

3. *Enjoy your delicious and varied meals!*

CHAPTER 4: DINNER DELICACIES

Baked Cod with Lemon and Dill

Time Frame:

Prep Time: 10 minutes

Cook Time: 15 minutes

Total Time: 25 minutes

Ingredients:

4 cod fillets

Salt and pepper to taste

2 tablespoons olive oil

2 tablespoons fresh lemon juice

1 tablespoon fresh dill, chopped

Lemon slices for garnish

Instructions:

Preheat the oven to 400°F (200°C) and line a baking sheet with parchment paper.

Place cod fillets on the prepared baking sheet. Season with salt and pepper.

Drizzle olive oil and lemon juice over the fillets, then sprinkle with chopped dill.

Bake for 12-15 minutes or until the fish is cooked through and flakes easily.

Garnish with lemon slices before serving.

Tips:

Serve with steamed vegetables or a side salad.

Adjust the seasoning and lemon to suit your taste.

Spaghetti Squash with Meatballs and Tomato Sauce

Time Frame:

Prep Time: 15 minutes

Cook Time: 45 minutes

Total Time: 1 hour

Ingredients:

1 medium spaghetti squash

1 pound ground meat (beef, turkey, or a mix)

1/2 cup breadcrumbs

1 egg

2 cups tomato sauce

Fresh basil for garnish

Grated Parmesan cheese (optional)

Instructions:

Preheat the oven to 400°F (200°C).

Cut the spaghetti squash in half, remove the seeds, and place it cut-side down on a baking sheet. Roast for 30-40 minutes or until the squash is fork-tender.

While the squash is roasting, mix ground meat, breadcrumbs, and egg. Form into meatballs.

In a skillet, brown the meatballs over medium heat. Add tomato sauce and simmer until meatballs are cooked through.

Once the spaghetti squash is done, use a fork to scrape the strands into a bowl.

Top the squash with meatballs and tomato sauce.

Garnish with fresh basil and Parmesan cheese if desired.

Tips:

Customize the meatballs with your favorite herbs and spices.

Use store-bought tomato sauce or make your own.

Stir-Fried Tofu with Low FODMAP Vegetables

Time Frame:

Prep Time: 15 minutes

Cook Time: 10 minutes

Total Time: 25 minutes

Ingredients:

1 block extra-firm tofu, pressed and cubed

2 tablespoons low FODMAP stir-fry sauce

1 tablespoon sesame oil

1 cup broccoli florets

1 bell pepper, sliced

1 zucchini, sliced

Green onions (green parts only) for garnish

Instructions:

Heat sesame oil in a wok or large skillet over medium-high heat.

Add cubed tofu and stir-fry until golden brown.

Add broccoli, bell pepper, and zucchini to the pan. Stir-fry for 3-5 minutes until vegetables are tender-crisp.

Pour low FODMAP stir-fry sauce over the tofu and vegetables. Stir well to coat.

Garnish with sliced green onions before serving.

Tips:

Choose low FODMAP vegetables like bell peppers, zucchini, and broccoli.

Serve over rice or rice noodles if desired.

Grilled Shrimp and Pineapple Skewers

Time Frame:

Prep Time: 20 minutes

Cook Time: 6 minutes

Total Time: 26 minutes

Ingredients:

1 pound large shrimp, peeled and deveined

1 cup pineapple chunks

2 tablespoons olive oil

1 tablespoon soy sauce

1 tablespoon honey

1 teaspoon grated ginger

Wooden skewers, soaked in water

Instructions:

Preheat the grill to medium-high heat.

In a bowl, whisk together olive oil, soy sauce, honey, and grated ginger.

Thread shrimp and pineapple chunks onto skewers, alternating.

Brush the skewers with the marinade.

Grill for 2-3 minutes per side or until shrimp are opaque and cooked through.

Tips:

Serve over rice or a bed of greens.

Add a sprinkle of sesame seeds for extra flavor.

Eggplant and Red Pepper Lasagna

Time Frame:

Prep Time: 30 minutes

Cook Time: 40 minutes

Total Time: 1 hour 10 minutes

Ingredients:

1 large eggplant, thinly sliced

2 red bell peppers, sliced

2 cups ricotta cheese

1 cup grated mozzarella cheese

1/2 cup grated Parmesan cheese

2 cups marinara sauce

Fresh basil for garnish

Salt and pepper to taste

Instructions:

Preheat the oven to 375°F (190°C).

Lightly salt eggplant slices and let them sit for 15 minutes to release excess moisture. Pat dry with paper towels.

In a baking dish, layer eggplant slices, red bell peppers, ricotta cheese, mozzarella cheese, Parmesan cheese, and marinara sauce.

Repeat the layers, finishing with a layer of marinara sauce and a sprinkle of Parmesan.

Bake for 35-40 minutes or until the lasagna is bubbly and golden.

Garnish with fresh basil before serving.

Tips:

Make sure to slice the eggplant thinly for even cooking.

Allow the lasagna to rest for a few minutes before serving.

Teriyaki Chicken with Sesame Green Beans

Time Frame:

Prep Time: 15 minutes

Cook Time: 15 minutes

Total Time: 30 minutes

Ingredients:

1 lb boneless, skinless chicken thighs, cut into bite-sized pieces

1/2 cup teriyaki sauce

2 tablespoons soy sauce

1 tablespoon honey

1 tablespoon sesame oil

1 lb green beans, trimmed

Sesame seeds for garnish

Cooked rice for serving

Instructions:

In a bowl, marinate chicken pieces in teriyaki sauce, soy sauce, honey, and sesame oil for at least 15 minutes.

Heat a large skillet over medium-high heat. Add marinated chicken and cook until browned and cooked through.

In a separate pot, steam or blanch green beans until crisp-tender.

Serve teriyaki chicken over cooked rice with sesame green beans on the side.

Garnish with sesame seeds before serving.

Tips:

Use low-sodium soy sauce for a healthier option.

Customize with your favorite vegetables in the stir-fry.

Enjoy preparing and savoring these delicious meals!

CHAPTER 5: SNACK ATTACK

Roasted Rosemary Almonds

Time Frame:

Prep Time: 5 minutes

Roasting Time: 15 minutes

Total Time: 20 minutes

Ingredients:

2 cups raw almonds

1 tablespoon olive oil

1 tablespoon fresh rosemary, chopped

Salt to taste

Instructions:

Preheat the oven to 350°F (175°C).

In a bowl, toss almonds with olive oil, chopped rosemary, and salt.

Spread the almonds in a single layer on a baking sheet.

Roast for 12-15 minutes, stirring halfway through.

Let the almonds cool before serving.

Tips:

Adjust the salt and rosemary to your preference.

Store in an airtight container for freshness.

Cucumber and Carrot Sticks with Hummus

Time Frame:

Prep Time: 10 minutes

Total Time: 10 minutes

Ingredients:

2 cucumbers, cut into sticks

4 carrots, cut into sticks

1 cup hummus

Instructions:

Wash and cut the cucumbers and carrots into stick shapes.

Arrange the vegetable sticks on a serving platter.

Serve with a bowl of hummus for dipping.

Tips:

Use baby carrots for convenience.

Experiment with different hummus flavors.

FODMAP-friendly Trail Mix

Time Frame:

Prep Time: 5 minutes

Total Time: 5 minutes

Ingredients:

1 cup mixed nuts (almonds, walnuts, pecans)

1 cup pumpkin seeds (pepitas)

1 cup dried blueberries

1/2 cup dark chocolate chips

Instructions:

In a bowl, mix together the nuts, pumpkin seeds, dried blueberries, and dark chocolate chips.

Toss well to combine.

Portion into individual snack bags for convenience.

Tips:

Choose FODMAP-friendly nuts and dried fruits.

Adjust the ratios based on personal preferences.

Baked Parmesan Zucchini Chips

Time Frame:

Prep Time: 15 minutes

Baking Time: 20 minutes

Total Time: 35 minutes

Ingredients:

2 medium zucchinis, thinly sliced

1/2 cup grated Parmesan cheese

1 teaspoon garlic powder

1 teaspoon dried oregano

Salt and pepper to taste

Olive oil spray

Instructions:

Preheat the oven to 425°F (220°C).

In a bowl, toss zucchini slices with Parmesan cheese, garlic powder, oregano, salt, and pepper.

Place the coated zucchini slices on a baking sheet lined with parchment paper.

Lightly spray the zucchini with olive oil.

Bake for 18-20 minutes or until the edges are golden brown and crisp.

Tips:

Use a mandoline slicer for consistent zucchini thickness.

Enjoy them immediately for the best crunch.

Strawberry and Cantaloupe Skewers

Time Frame:

Prep Time: 15 minutes

Total Time: 15 minutes

Ingredients:

Fresh strawberries, hulled

Cantaloupe, cut into cubes

Wooden skewers

Instructions:

Alternate threading strawberries and cantaloupe cubes onto wooden skewers.

Arrange the skewers on a serving platter.

Tips:

Chill the skewers in the refrigerator before serving for a refreshing treat.

Drizzle with honey for extra sweetness.

Rice Cake with Peanut Butter and Banana Slices

Time Frame:

Prep Time: 5 minutes

Total Time: 5 minutes

Ingredients:

Rice cakes

Peanut butter (or almond butter for variety)

Banana, sliced

Instructions:

Spread a layer of peanut butter on each rice cake.

Top with banana slices.

Tips:

Choose whole-grain rice cakes for added fiber.

Sprinkle with chia seeds or cinnamon for extra flavor.

These recipes make for delicious and healthy snacks. Enjoy!

CONCLUSION

In conclusion, "Low FODMAP Cookbook for Beginners: 1200+ Simple and Delicious Recipes to Calm Your Guts and Combat Digestive Issues" stands as an invaluable resource for individuals seeking not only relief from digestive issues but also a journey towards a healthier and more enjoyable relationship with food. As we delve into the final chapters of this culinary guide, it becomes evident that the impact of the low FODMAP diet extends far beyond the mere management of gastrointestinal discomfort; it is a transformative approach to eating that empowers individuals to take charge of their well-being.

The author's meticulous attention to detail, backed by a comprehensive understanding of the low FODMAP framework, makes this cookbook a standout guide in the realm of digestive health. The inclusion of over 1200 recipes ensures that there is a wealth of options catering to various tastes, preferences, and dietary requirements. From breakfast to dinner, snacks to desserts, the cookbook provides a diverse array of dishes that not only adhere to the low FODMAP principles but also burst with flavor and creativity.

One of the commendable aspects of this book is its accessibility. The author skillfully breaks down the sometimes complex low FODMAP concept into easily understandable segments, making it approachable for both beginners and seasoned cooks alike. The incorporation of practical tips, meal plans, and shopping lists further enhances the user-friendly nature of the cookbook, facilitating a seamless transition into the low FODMAP lifestyle.

Beyond the realm of recipes, the book offers a wealth of information on the science behind the low FODMAP diet. The reader gains insights into the intricacies of how certain fermentable carbohydrates can trigger digestive discomfort and how strategic food choices can alleviate these symptoms. This scientific foundation adds depth to the cookbook, allowing readers to make informed decisions about their dietary habits.

As we navigate through the pages of this cookbook, it becomes evident that the author not only aims to provide a collection of recipes but also strives to foster a sense of empowerment and autonomy in the readers. The cookbook encourages a mindful and intentional approach to eating, challenging individuals to be more attuned to their bodies and the impact of food on their overall well-being.

Furthermore, the inclusion of personal anecdotes, success stories, and testimonials from individuals who have benefited from the low FODMAP approach adds a human touch to the book. It instills a sense of hope and reassurance for those embarking on this dietary journey, reminding them that they are not alone in their quest for digestive health.

In the grand tapestry of health and wellness literature, the "Low FODMAP Cookbook for Beginners" distinguishes itself as a beacon of practical guidance and culinary inspiration. It is not merely a compilation of recipes but a holistic guide that equips individuals with the knowledge, tools, and motivation to transform their relationship with food and reclaim control over their digestive health. As readers close the pages of this cookbook, they are not just armed with recipes but with a newfound sense of empowerment and the promise of a healthier and more vibrant life.